AMERICAN M

AMERICAN
MEDICINAL LEAVES
AND HERBS

US DEPARTMENT OF AGRICULTURE
BULLETIN 219

First Edition 1911
Alice Henkel

New Edition 2020
Edited by Tarl Warwick

Illustrations by Rita Metzner

1

COPYRIGHT AND DISCLAIMER

FOREWORD

This little handbook is one of the greater herbal works of its era, supplying a list of fully illustrated medicinally active species by the dozen, all nicely compiled by the USDA itself.

While the use of herbs in medicine has largely fallen out of favor, replaced by synthetic drugs and fully modern chemistry, we must understand that the organic compounds extracted from plants, fungi, and other sources were the best that could be obtained a century ago and, even today, remain in use in the undeveloped world and among homeopathic groups.

The list of species here is substantial; Wintergreen, spearmint, and many others are still used today in the context of cooking at least and as flavorful additives to many recipes. Some I have tried personally; bearberry liquor (sold under the moniker of "crowberry" in Iceland) is delicious. A few species- such as jimson weed (Datura Stramonium) are normally avoided now because they are substantially harmful if administered improperly.

This edition of "American Medicinal Leaves and Herbs" has been carefully edited for format and content. Care has been taken to retain all original intent and meaning.

AMERICAN MEDICINAL LEAVES AND HERBS

LETTER OF TRANSMITTAL.
U. S. DEPARTMENT OF AGRICULTURE
BUREAU OF PLANT INDUSTRY
OFFICE OF THE CHIEF

Washington, D. C., April 15, 1911.

SIR: I have the honor to transmit herewith and to recommend for publication as Bulletin No. 219 of the series of this Bureau the accompanying manuscript, entitled "American Medicinal Leaves and Herbs." This paper was prepared by Miss Alice Henkel, Assistant in Drug-Plant Investigations, and has been submitted by the Physiologist in charge with a view to its publication.

Thirty-six plants furnishing leaves and herbs for medicinal use are fully described, and in some instances brief descriptions of related species are included therewith. Of the above number, 15 are official in the United States Pharmacopoeia. This bulletin forms the third installment on the subject of American medicinal plants and has been prepared to meet the steady demand for information of this character. It is intended as a guide and reference book for those who may be interested in the study or collection of the medicinal plants of this country. The first bulletin of this series treats of American root drugs, and the second of American medicinal barks.

Respectfully,
WM. A. TAYLOR,
Acting Chief of Bureau.
Hon. JAMES WILSON,
Secretary of Agriculture.

AMERICAN MEDICINAL LEAVES AND HERBS

INTRODUCTION

Less difficulty will be encountered in the collection of leaves and herbs than in the case of other portions of plants, for not only is recognition easier, since, especially in the matter of herbs, these parts are usually gathered at a time when the plants are in flower, but the labor is less arduous, for there are no roots to dig or barks to peel. Of the three dozen medicinal plants mentioned in this bulletin, 15 are recognized as official in the Eighth Decennial Revision of the United States Pharmacopoeia. This is more than half of all the leaves and herbs included in the Pharmacopoeia.

Among the plants included in this bulletin are peppermint and spearmint, which are found not only in the wild state but the cultivation of which for the distillation of the oil constitutes an important American industry. Especially is this true of peppermint? Thousands of acres being devoted to the cultivation of this plant, principally in the States of Michigan and New York. A number of other plants mentioned in this paper furnish useful oils, such as oil of wintergreen, pennyroyal, fleabane, tansy, wormwood, and fire-weed.

As in the case of other bulletins of this series, an effort has been made to include in it only such plants as seem most in demand, lack of space forbidding a consideration of others which are or have been used to a more limited extent. With two or three exceptions the illustrations have been reproduced from photographs taken from nature by Mr. C. L. Lochman.

COLLECTION OF LEAVES AND HERBS

Leaves are usually collected when they have attained full

development and may be obtained by cutting off the entire plant and stripping the leaves from the stem, using a scythe to mow the plants where they occur in sufficient abundance to warrant this, or the leaves may be picked from the plants as they grow in the field. Whenever the plants are cut down in quantity they must be carefully looked over afterwards for the purpose of sorting out such other plants as may have been accidentally cut with them. Stems should be discarded as much as possible, and where a leaf is composed of several leaflets these are usually detached from the stems.

In gathering herbs only the flowering tops and leaves and the more tender stems should be taken, the coarse and large stems being rejected. All withered, diseased, or discolored portions should be removed from both leaves and herbs.

In order that they may retain their bright-green color and characteristic odor after drying, leaves and herbs must be carefully dried in the shade, allowing the air to circulate freely but keeping out all moisture; dampness will darken them, and they must therefore be placed under cover at night or in rainy weather. A bright color is desirable, as such a product will sell more readily. To dry them the leaves and herbs should be spread out thinly on clean racks or shelves and turned frequently until thoroughly dry. They readily absorb moisture and when perfectly cured should be stored in a dry place.

Leaves and herbs generally become very brittle when they are dry and must be very carefully packed to cause as little crushing as possible. They should be firmly packed in sound burlap or gunny sacks or in dry, clean boxes or barrels. Before shipping the goods, however, good-sized representative samples of the leaves and herbs to be disposed of should be sent to drug dealers for their inspection, together with a letter stating how large a quantity the collector has to sell.

AMERICAN MEDICINAL LEAVES AND HERBS

With the changes in prices that are constantly taking place in the drug market it is, of course, impossible to give definite prices in this paper, and only approximate quotations are therefore included in order that the collector may form some idea concerning the possible range of prices. Only through correspondence with drug dealers can the actual price then prevailing be ascertained.

PLANTS FURNISHING MEDICINAL LEAVES AND HERBS

Each section contains synonyms, the pharmacopoeial name (if any), the common names, habitat, range, descriptions, and information concerning the collection, prices, and uses of the plants. The medicinal uses are referred to in a general way only, since it is not within the province of a publication of this kind to give detailed information in regard to such matters. Advice concerning the proper remedies to use should be sought only from physicians. The statements made in this paper as to medicinal uses are based on information contained in various dispensatories and other works relating to materia medica.

SWEET FERN

Comptonia peregrina (L.) Coulter.

Synonyms: Comptonia asplenifolia Gaertn.; Myrica asplenifolia L.; Liquidambar asplenifolia L.; Liquidambar peregrina L.

Other common names: Fern gale, fern bush, meadow fern, shrubby fern, Canada sweet gale, spleenwort bush, sweet bush, sweet ferry.

Habitat and range: Sweet fern is usually found on hillsides, in dry soil, in Canada and the northeastern United States. It is indigenous.

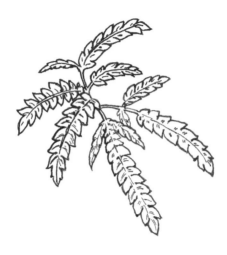

Fig. 1: Sweet Fern.

Description: The fragrant odor and. the resemblance of the leaves of this plant to those of a fern have given rise to the common name "sweet fern." It is a shrub with reddish-brown bark, growing from about 1 to 3 feet in height, with slender, erect or spreading branches, the leaves hairy when young. The thin narrow leaves are borne on short stalks and are linear oblong or linear lance shaped, about 3 to 6 inches long and from one-fourth to half an inch wide, deeply divided into many lobes, the margins of which are generally entire or sparingly toothed. The catkins expand with the leaves. (Fig. 1.)

The staminate or male flowers are produced in cylindrical catkins in clusters at the ends of the branches and are about an inch in length, the kidney-shaped scales overlapping. The pistillate or female flowers are borne in egg-shaped or roundish-oval catkins, the eight awl-shaped bractlets persisting and surrounding the one-seeded, shining, light brown nut, giving it a burlike appearance. The whole plant has a spicy, aromatic odor, which is more pronounced when the leaves are bruised.

Sweet fern belongs to the bayberry family (Myricaceae).

Collection, prices, and uses: The entire plant is used, but especially the leaves and tops. It has a fragrant, spicy odor and an aromatic, slightly bitter, and astringent taste. The present price of sweet fern is about 3 to 5 cents a pound. It is used for its tonic and astringent properties, principally in a domestic way, as a remedy in diarrheal complaints.

LIVERLEAF

(1) *Hepatica hepatica* (L.) Karst.; (2) *Hepatica acuta* (Pursh) Britton.

Synonyms: (1) Hepatica triloba Chaix.; Anemone hepatica L. (2) Hepatica triloba var. acuta Pursh; Hepatica acutiloba DC.

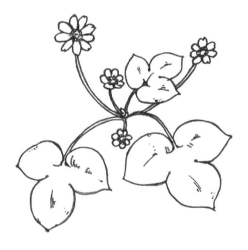

Fig. 2: Liverleaf

AMERICAN MEDICINAL LEAVES AND HERBS

Other common names: (1) Round-leaved hepatica, common liverleaf, kidney liver-leaf, liverwort (incorrect), noble liverwort, heart liverwort, three-leaved liverwort, liverweed, herb-trinity, golden trefoil, ivy flower, mouse-ears, squirrel cup; (2) heart liverleaf, acute-lobed liverleaf, sharp-lobed liverleaf, sharp-lobed hepatica.

Habitat and range: The common liverleaf is found in woods from Nova Scotia to northern Florida and west to Iowa and Missouri, while the heart liverleaf occurs from Quebec to Ontario, south to Georgia (but rare near the coast), and west to Iowa and Minnesota.

Description: The hepaticas are among the earliest of our spring flowers, blossoming about March, and frequently before that time. They grow only about 4 to 6 inches in height, with leaves produced from the roots on long soft-hairy stalks and spreading on the ground. The thick and leathery evergreen leaves are kidney shaped or roundish and deeply divided into three oval, blunt lobes; the young leaves are pale green and soft hairy, but the older ones become leathery and smooth, expanding. when mature to almost 3 inches across; they are dark green above, sometimes with a purplish tinge, and also of a purplish color on the under surface. The flowers, which are about one-half inch in diameter, are borne singly on slender, hairy stalks arising from the root, and vary in color from bluish to purple or white. Immediately beneath the flower are three small, stemless, oval, and blunt leaflets or bracts, which are thickly covered with soft, silky hairs. (Fig. 2.) The heart liverleaf is very similar to the common liverleaf. It grows perhaps a trifle taller and the lobes of the leaf and the small leaflets or bracts immediately under the flower are more sharply pointed.

The hepaticas are members of the crowfoot family (Ranunculacese) and are perennials. The name "liverwort," often given to these plants, is incorrect, since it belongs to an entirely different genus.

Collection, prices, and uses: The leaves, which were official in the United States Pharmacopoeia from 1830 to 1880, are the parts employed; they should be collected in April. They lose about three fourths of their weight in drying. The price at present paid for them is about 4 to 5 cents a pound. Liverleaf is employed for its tonic properties and is said to be useful in affections of the liver.

CELANDINE

Chelidonium majus L.

Other common names: Chelidonium, garden celandine, greater celandine, tetter-wort, killwart, wart flower, wartweed, wartwort, felonwort, cockfoot. devil's-milk, Jacob's ladder, swallow-wort, wretweed.

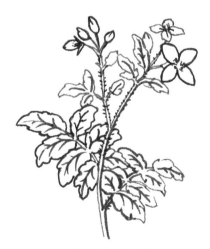

Fig. 3: Celandine

Habitat and range: Celandine, naturalized from Europe, is found in rich damp soil along fences and roadsides near towns from Maine to Ontario and southward. It is common from southern Maine to Pennsylvania.

Description: This plant, which has rather weak, brittle stems arising from a reddish brown, branching root, is a biennial belonging to the poppy family (Papaveraceae) and, like other members of this family, contains an acrid juice, which in this species is colored yellow. It is an erect, branched, sparingly hairy herb, from about 1 to 2 feet in height with thin leaves 4 to 8 inches in length. The leaves, which are lyre shaped in outline, are deeply and variously cleft, the lobes thus formed being oval, blunt, and wavy or round toothed, or rather deeply cut. They have a grayish-green appearance, especially on the lower surface.

The small, 4-petaled, sulfur-yellow flowers of the celandine are produced from about April to September, followed by smooth, long, pod-shaped capsules crowned with the persistent style and stigma and containing numerous seeds. (Fig. 3.)

Collection, prices, and uses: The entire plant, which was official in the United States Pharmacopoeia for 1890, is used. It should be collected when the herb is in flower. At present it brings about 6 or 8 cents a pound. The fresh plant has an unpleasant, acrid odor when bruised, but in the dried state it is odorless. It has a persistent acrid and somewhat salty taste. Celandine is an old remedy. It has cathartic and diuretic properties, promotes perspiration, and has been used as an expectorant. The juice has been employed externally for warts, corns, and some forms of skin diseases.

WITCH HAZEL

Hamamelis virginiana L.

Pharmacopoeial name: Hamamelidis folia.

Other common names: Snapping hazel, winterbloom, wych-hazel, striped alder, spotted alder, tobacco wood.

Habitat and range: The home of this native shrub is in low damp woods from New Brunswick to Minnesota and south to Florida and Texas.

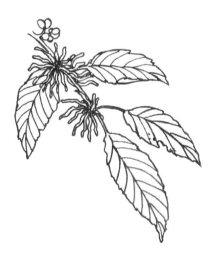

Fig. 4 Witch-Hazel

Description: This shrub, while it may grow to 25 feet in height, is more frequently found reaching a height of only 8 to 15 feet, its crooked stem and long forking branches covered with smoothish brown bark sometimes with an addition of lichens. A peculiar feature about witch hazel is its flowering in very late fall

13

or even early winter, when its branches are destitute of leaves, the seed forming but not ripening until the following season. The leaves are rather large, 3 to 5 inches long, thick, and borne on short stalks; they are broadly oval or heart-shaped oval, sometimes pointed and sometimes blunt at the apex, with uneven sides at the base, and wavy margins. The older leaves are smooth, but when young they are covered with downy hairs. The upper surface of the leaves is a light-green or brownish green color, while the lower surface is pale green and somewhat shining, with prominent veins. The threadlike bright yellow flowers, which appear very late in autumn, are rather odd looking and consist of a 4-parted corolla with four long, narrow, strap-shaped petals, which are twisted in various ways when in full flower. The seed capsule does not mature until the following season, when the beaked and densely hairy seed case bursts open elastically, scattering with great force and to a considerable distance the large, shining-black, hard seeds. (Fig. 4.) This interesting shrub is a member of the witch-hazel family (Hamamelidaceae).

Collection, prices, and uses: Witch-hazel leaves are official in the United States Pharmacopoeia. They should be collected in autumn and carefully dried. Formerly the leaves alone were recognized in the United States Pharmacopoeia, but now the bark and twigs are also official. The leaves have a faint odor and an astringent, somewhat bitter, and aromatic taste. They bring about 2 to 3 cents a pound. The soothing properties of witch-hazel were known among the Indians, and it is still employed for the relief of inflammatory conditions.

AMERICAN SENNA

Cassia marilandica L.

Synonym: Senna marilandica (Link.)

14

AMERICAN MEDICINAL LEAVES AND HERBS

Other common names: Wild senna, locust plant.

Habitat and range: American senna generally frequents wet or swampy soils from New England to North Carolina and westward to Louisiana and Nebraska.

Description: This is a native species, a member of the senna family (Caesalpiniaceae), which is closely related to the pea family. It is a perennial herb, its round grooved stems reaching about 4 to 6 feet in height. The leaves, which are borne on long, somewhat bristly hairy stalks, are 6 to 8 inches long and consist of from 12 to 20 leaflets placed opposite to each other on the stem. Each leaflet is oblong or lance-shaped oblong, blunt at the top but terminating with a short, stiff point, rounded at the base and from 1 to 10 inches long, the stalks supporting them being rather short; the upper surface is of a pale-green color, while underneath it is still lighter in color and covered with a bloom. On the upper surface of the leaf stem, near its base, is a prominent club-shaped gland, borne on a stalk.

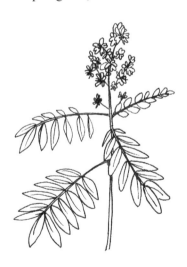

Fig.5 : American Senna

The numerous yellow flowers are borne on slender, hairy stems, produced in clusters in the axils of the leaves at the top of the plant and appearing from about August to September. The pods are about 3 inches in length, linear, somewhat curved and drooping, slightly hairy at first, flat, and narrowed on the sides between the seeds. They contain numerous small, flat, dark-brown seeds. (Fig. 5.)

Collection, prices, and uses: The leaves, or rather the leaflets, are the parts employed and should be gathered at flowering time, which usually occurs during July and August. They were official in the United States Pharmacopoeia from 1820 to 1880. American senna leaves have a very slight odor and a rather disagreeable taste, somewhat like that of the foreign senna. It is used for purposes similar to the well-known senna of commerce imported from abroad, having, like that, cathartic properties. The price at present paid for American senna is about 6 to 8 cents a pound.

EVENING PRIMROSE

Oenothera biennis L.

Synonyms: Onagra biennis (L.) Scop.; Oenothera muricata L.

Other common names: Common evening primrose, wild evening primrose, field evening primrose, tree primrose, fever plant, night willow-herb, king's cure-all, large rampion, scurvish, scabish.

Habitat and range: This is a widely distributed herb, its range extending from Labrador south to Florida and west to the Rocky Mountains. It usually frequents fields and waste places, occurring in dry soil.

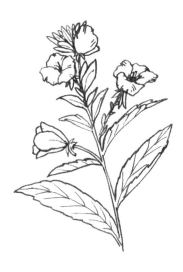

Fig. 6: Evening Primrose

Description: The evening primrose is a coarse annual or biennial weed, which has the peculiarity that its flowers do not open until evening, remaining open all night and closing the next morning, but not expanding again. It is generally stout and erect in growth, from 1 foot to about 5 feet in height, simple or branched, usually hairy and leafy. The leaves are 1 to 6 inches in length, lance shaped and sharp pointed at the top, with wavy toothed margins narrowing toward the base. With the exception of some of the leaves near the base, most of them are stemless. The spikes of fragrant sulfur-yellow flowers are produced from about June to October and, as already stated and as indicated by the name "evening" primrose, they are open late in the evening and during the night. They are borne at the end of the stem and are interspersed with leafy bracts. Each flower has four spreading petals and measures about 1 to 2 inches across. The seed capsules are oblong and hairy, about an inch in length, and narrowed at the top. (Fig. 6.) This plant belongs to the evening primrose family (Onagraceae).

Collection, prices, and uses: The entire plant is used. It is collected about flowering time, bringing about 5 cents a pound. The herb has a somewhat astringent and mucilaginous taste, but no odor. It has been used for coughs and asthmatic troubles, and an ointment made therefrom has been employed as an application in skin affections.

YERBA SANTA

Eriodictyon californicum (H. and A.) Greene.

Pharmacopoeial name: Eriodictyon.

Synonym: Eriodictyon glutinosum Benth.

Other common names: Mountain balm, consumptive's weed, bear's weed, gum plant, tarweed.

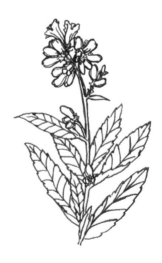

Fig. 7: Yerba Santa

Description: This evergreen shrub, a member of the waterleaf family (Hydrophyllaceae), reaches a height of from 3 to 4 feet, bearing glutinous leaves. The stem is smooth, but exudes a gummy substance. The dark-green leaves are from 3 to 4 inches in length, placed alternately on the stem, oblong or oval lance shaped, leathery, narrowing gradually into a short stalk, and with margins generally toothed, except perhaps at the base: the upper surface is smooth, with depressed veins, the prominent veins on the under surface forming a strong network and the spaces between the veins covered with short felty hairs, giving it a white appearance. The leaves are coated with a resinous substance, making them appear as if varnished. The rather showy whitish or pale-blue flowers are borne in clusters at the top of the plant, the tubular, funnel-shaped corolla measuring about half an inch in length and having five spreading lobes. (Fig. 7.) The seed capsule is oval, grayish brown, and contains small, reddish-brown, shriveled seeds.

Collection, prices, and uses: The leaves are the parts collected for medicinal use and are official in the United States Pharmacopoeia. The price paid for them is about 5 cents a pound. Yerba santa has expectorant properties and is employed for throat and bronchial affections. It is also used as a bitter tonic. The odor is aromatic and the taste balsamic and sweetish.

PIPSISSEWA

Chimaphila umbellata (L.) Nutt.

Pharmacopoeial name: Chimaphila.

Synonyms: Pyrola umbellata L.; Chimaphila corymbosa Pursh.

Other common names: Prince's pine, pyrola, rheumatism

weed, bitter wintergreen, ground holly, king's cure, love-in-winter, noble pine, pine tulip.

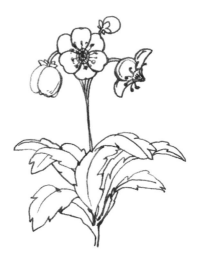

Fig. 8: Pipsissewa

Habitat and range: Pipsissewa is a native of this country, growing in dry, shady woods, especially in pine forests, and its range extends from Nova Scotia to British Columbia, south to Georgia, Mexico, and California. It also occurs in Europe and Asia.

Description: This small perennial herb, a foot or less in height, has a long, running, partly underground stem. It belongs to the heath family (Ericaceae) and has shining evergreen leaves of a somewhat leathery texture placed in a circle around the stem, usually near the top or scattered along it. They are dark green, broader at the top, with a sharp or blunt apex, narrowing toward the base and with margins sharply toothed; they are from about 1 to 2 inches long and about three-eighths to a little more than half an inch wide at the broadest part. From about June to August the pipsissewa may be found in flower, its pretty waxy-white or pinkish fragrant flowers, consisting of five rounded, concave petals, each one with a dark-pink spot at the base, nodding in clusters from the top of the erect stem. The brown capsules contain numerous very small seeds. (Fig. 8.)

Collection, prices, and uses: Although the United States Pharmacopoeia directs that the leaves be used, the entire plant is frequently employed, as all parts of it are active. Pipsissewa leaves have no odor, but a bitter, astringent taste. They bring about 4 cents a pound. Pipsissewa has slightly tonic, astringent, and diuretic properties and is sometimes employed in rheumatic and kidney affections. Externally it has been applied to ulcers.

Another species: The leaves of the spotted wintergreen (Chimaphila maculata Pursh) were official in the Pharmacopoeia of the United States from 1830 to 1840. These may be distinguished from the leaves of C. umbellata (pipsissewa) by their olive-green color marked with white along the midrib and veins. They are lance shaped in outline and are broadest at the base instead of at the top as in C. umbellata.

MOUNTAIN LAUREL

Kalmia latifolia L.

Other common names: Broad-leaved laurel, broad-leaved kalmia, American laurel, sheep laurel, rose laurel, spurge laurel, small laurel, wood laurel, kalmia, calico bush, spoonwood, spoon-hunt, ivy bush, bigleaved ivy, wicky, calmoun.

Habitat and range: The mountain laurel is found in sandy or rocky soil in woods from New Brunswick south to Ohio, Florida, and Louisiana.

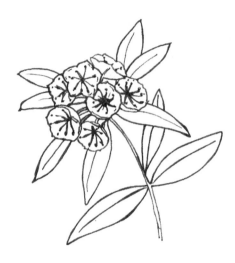

Fig. 9: Mountain Laurel

Description: This is an evergreen shrub from about 4 to 20 feet in height, with leathery leaves, and when in flower it is one of the most beautiful and showy of our native plants. It has very stiff branches and leathery oval or elliptical leaves borne on stems, mostly alternate, pointed at both ends, with margins entire, smooth and bright green on both sides, and having terminal, clammy-hairy clusters of flowers, which appear from about May to June. The buds are rather oddly shaped and fluted, at first of a deep rose color, expanding into saucer-shaped, more delicately tinted, whitish-pink flowers. Each saucer-shaped flower is provided with 10 pockets holding the anthers of the stamens, but from which these free themselves elastically when the flower is fully expanded. (Fig. 9.) The seed capsule is somewhat globular, the calyx and threadlike style remaining attached until the capsules open. Mountain laurel, which belongs to the heath family (Ericaceae), is poisonous to sheep and calves.

Collection, prices, and uses: The leaves, which bring about 3 to 4 cents a pound, are collected in the fall. They are used for their astringent properties.

GRAVEL PLANT

Epigaea repens L.

Other common names: Trailing arbutus, Mayflower, shad-flower, ground laurel, mountain pink, winter pink.

Habitat and range: This shrubby little plant spreads out on the ground in sandy soil, being found especially under evergreen trees from Florida to Michigan and northward.

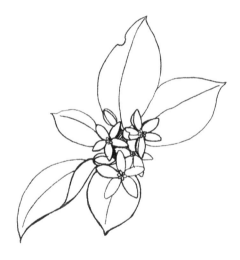

Fig. 10: Gravel Plant

Description: The gravel plant is one of our early spring flowers, and under its more popular name "trailing arbutus" it is greatly prized on account of its delicate shell-pink, waxy blossoms with their faint yet spicy fragrance. Gravel plant is the name that is generally applied to it in the drug trade. It spreads on the ground with stems 6 inches or more in length and has rust colored hairy twigs bearing evergreen leaves. The leaves are green above and below, thick and leathery, oval or roundish, sometimes with. the top pointed, blunt, or having a short stiff point and a rounded or heart-shaped base. The margins are unbroken and the upper surface is smooth, while the lower surface is somewhat hairy. The leaves measure from 1 to 3 inches in length and are about half as wide, the hairy stalks supporting them ranging from one-fourth of an inch to 2 inches in length. Early in the year, from about March to May, the flower clusters appear. These are borne in the axils of the leaves and at the ends of the branches and consist of several waxy, pinkish-white, fragrant flowers with saucer-shaped, 5-lobed corolla, the throat of the corolla tube being very densely hairy within. (Fig. 10.) The seed capsule is somewhat roundish, flattened, five celled, and contains numerous seeds. The gravel plant, belongs to the heath family (Ericaceae) and is a perennial.

Collection, prices, and uses: The leaves are collected at flowering time and are worth about 3 or 4 cents a pound. They have a bitter, astringent taste and are said to possess astringent and diuretic properties.

WINTERGREEN

Gaultheria procumbens L.

Other common names: Gaultheria, spring wintergreen, creeping wintergreen, aromatic wintergreen, spicy wintergreen, checkerberry, teaberry, partridge berry, grouseberry, spiceberry, chickenberry, deerberry, groundberry, hillberry, ivyberry, boxberry, redberry tea, Canadian tea, mountain tea, ivory plum, chinks, drunkards, red pollom, rapper dandies, wax cluster.

Habitat and range: This small native perennial frequents

sandy soils in cool damp woods, occurring especially under evergreen trees in Canada and the northeastern United States.

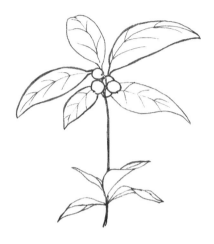

Fig. 11: Wintergreen

Description: Wintergreen is an aromatic, evergreen plant with an underground or creeping stem producing erect branches not more than 6 inches in height, the lower part of which is smooth and naked, while near the ends are borne the crowded clusters of evergreen leaves. These are alternate, shining dark green above, lighter colored underneath, spicy, thick and leathery, oval and narrowing toward the base, 1 to 1 1/2 inches in length, and of varying width. From about June to September the solitary, somewhat urn-shaped and five-toothed white and waxy flowers appear, borne on recurved stems in the axils of the leaves. (Fig. 11.) These are followed by globular, somewhat flattened berries, which ripen in autumn and remain on the plant, sometimes until spring. They are bright red, five celled, mealy, and spicy. All parts of the plant, which belongs to the heath family (Ericaceae), are aromatic.

Collection, prices, and uses: The leaves of wintergreen, or gaultheria, were at one time official in the United States Pharmacopoeia, but now only the oil of wintergreen, distilled from the leaves, is so regarded. The leaves should be collected in autumn. Sometimes the entire plant is pulled up and, after drying, the leaves readily shake off. The price paid to collectors ranges from about 3 to 4 cents a pound. Wintergreen has stimulant, antiseptic, and diuretic properties. Its chief use, however, seems to be as a flavoring agent.

BEARBERRY

Arctostaphylos uva-ursi (L.) Spreng.

Pharmacopoeial name: Uva ursi.

Other common names: Red bearberry, bear's-grape, bear's bilberry, bear's whortleberry, foxberry, upland cranberry, mountain cranberry, crowberry, mealberry, rock-berry, mountain box, kinnikinnic, killikinic, universe vine, brawlins, burren myrtle, creashak, sagachomi, rapper dandies (fruit).

Habitat and range: Bearberry is a native of this country, growing in dry sandy or rocky soil from the Middle Atlantic States north to Labrador and westward to California and Alaska.

Description: The bearberry is a low, much-branched shrub trailing over the ground and having leathery, evergreen leaves. It is a member of the heath family (Ericaceae) and produces its pretty waxy flowers about May. The numerous crowded leaves are thick and leathery, evergreen, about one-half to 1 inch in length, blunt and widest at the top and narrowing at the base, with a network of fine veins, smooth, and with margins entire. The flowers are few, borne in short drooping clusters at the ends of the branches, and are ovoid or somewhat bell shaped

26

in form, four or five lobed, white with a pinkish tinge. They are followed by smooth, red, globular fruits, with an insipid, rather dry pulp, containing five nutlets. (Fig. 12.)

Fig. 12: Bearberry

Collection, prices, and uses: Bearberry or uva ursi leaves, official in the United States Pharmacopoeia, are collected in autumn. Collectors receive from about 2 to 4 cents a pound for them. Bearberry leaves have a bitter, astringent taste and a faint odor. They act on the kidneys and bladder and have astringent and tonic properties.

Another species: The leaves of manzanita (Arctostaphylos glauca Lindl.), a shrub-like tree, 9 to 25 feet high, have properties similar to uva ursi and are also used in medicine for similar purposes. They are of a leathery texture, pale green, ovate oblong in shape, with unbroken margins, and about 2 inches in length. Manzanita grows in California, in dry rocky districts on the western slopes of the Sierras.

BUCK BEAN

Menyanthes trifoliata L.

Other common names: Bog bean, bog myrtle, bog hop, bog nut, brook bean, bean trefoil, marsh trefoil, water trefoil, bitter trefoil, water shamrock, marsh clover, moonflower, bitterworm.

Habitat and range: The buck bean is a marsh herb occurring in North America as far south as Pennsylvania, Minnesota, and California. It is also native in Europe.

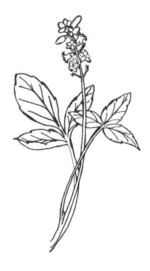

Fig. 13: Buck bean

Description: This perennial herb arises from a long, black, creeping, scaly rootstock, the leaves being produced from the end of the same on erect sheathing stems measuring about 2 to 10 inches in height. The leaves consist of three oblong-oval or broadly oval leaflets 11/2 to 3 inches long, somewhat fleshy and smooth, blunt at the top, with margins entire and narrowed toward the base; the upper surface is pale green and the lower surface somewhat glossy, with the thick midrib light in color. The flower cluster is produced from May to July on a long, thick, naked stalk arising from the rootstock It bears from 10 to 20 flowers, each with a funnel-shaped tube terminating in five segments which are pinkish purple or whitish on the outside and whitish and thickly bearded with white hairs within. (Fig. 13.) The capsules which follow are ovate, blunt at the top, smooth and light brown, and contain numerous smooth and shining seeds. Buck bean is a perennial belonging to the buck-bean family (Menyanthaceae).

Collection, prices, and uses: The leaves are generally collected in spring. They lose more than three-fourths of their weight in drying. The price paid per pound is about 6 to 8 cents. Buck-bean leaves have a very bitter taste, but no odor. Large doses are said to have cathartic and sometimes emetic action, but the principal use of buck-bean leaves is as a bitter tonic. They have been employed in dyspepsia, fevers, rheumatic and skin affections, and also as a remedy against worms. The rootstock is also sometimes employed medicinally and was recognized in the United States Pharmacopoeia from 1830 to 1840.

SKULLCAP

Scutellaria lateriflora L.

Pharmacopoeial name: Scutellaria.

Other common names: American skullcap, blue skullcap, mad-dog skullcap, side-flowering skullcap, madweed, hoodwort, blue pimpernel, hooded willow-herb.

Habitat and range: This species is native in damp places

29

along banks of streams from Canada southward to Florida, New Mexico, and Washington.

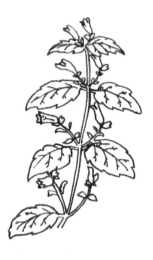

Fig. 14: Skullcap

Description: The lip-shaped flowers and squarish stems of the skullcap indicate that it is a member of the mint family (Menthaceae). It is a perennial of slender, erect habit, its square, leafy, branching stem ranging from 8 inches to 2 feet in height, smooth, or sometimes hairy at the top. The leaves are placed opposite to each other on the stem on slender stalks and are about 1 to 3 inches in length and about one-third as wide, thin in texture, oblong or lance shaped, with margins coarsely toothed. They gradually become smaller toward the top, and sometimes those at the very top have the margins unbroken. The flowers are borne in narrow, spikelike, one-sided clusters, generally in the axils of the leaves, but frequently also at the top, and are interspersed with leafy bracts. They appear from about July to September and are blue, shading off to whitish. The tubular, 2-lipped flowers are about a quarter of an inch in length, and the calyx, or outer green covering of the flower, is also two lipped,

30

the upper lip shaped like a helmet and closing in fruit. (Fig. 14.)

Collection, prices, and uses: The dried plant is at present official in the United States Pharmacopoeia. The entire plant is collected when in flower and should be carefully dried in the shade. The price ranges from about 3 to 4 cents a pound. Very frequently collectors will gather some other species in place of the official plant, most of those thus wrongly finding their way into the market being generally of stouter growth, with broader leaves and much larger flowers. This plant was once considered valuable for the prevention of hydrophobia, whence the names "mad-dog skullcap" and "madweed," but it is now known to be useless for that purpose. It is used principally as a tonic and to a limited extent for allaying nervous irritation of various kinds.

HOREHOUND

Marrubium vulgare L.

Pharmacopoial name: Marrubium.

Other common names: Houndsbene, marvel, marrube.

Habitat and range: Horehound grows in dry sandy or stony soil in waste places, along roadsides and near dwellings, in fields, and pastures. It is found from Maine to South Carolina, Texas, and westward to California and Oregon. It is very abundant in pastures in Oregon and California, and especially in southern California, where it is a very trouble-some weed, covering vast areas and in such dense masses as to crowd out all other vegetation. It has been naturalized from Europe.

Description: The entire plant is thickly covered with hairs, which give it a whitish, woolly appearance. It is a bushy, branching herb, having a pleasant aromatic odor, and is about 1 to 3 feet high, with many woolly stems rounded below and four angled above, with opposite, oval or roundish, wrinkled, strongly veined, and very hoary leaves. The leaves are about 1 to 2 inches in length, placed opposite each other on the stem, oval or nearly round, somewhat blunt at the apex, and narrowed or somewhat heart shaped at the base, the margins round toothed; the upper surface is wrinkled and somewhat hairy, while the lower surface is very hoary and prominently veined. The lip-shaped flowers, which appear from June to September, show that it is a member of the mint family (Menthaceae). These are borne in dense woolly clusters in the axils of the leaves and are whitish, two lipped, the upper lip two lobed, the lower three lobed. The hooked calyx teeth of the mature flower heads cling to the wool of sheep, resulting in the scattering of the seeds. (Fig. 15.)

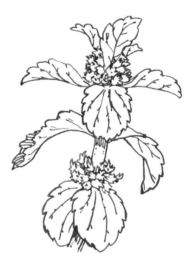

Fig. 15: Horehound

Collection, prices, and uses: The leaves and tops are the parts used in medicine and are official in the United States Pharmacopoeia. These are gathered just before the plant is in flower, the coarse stalks being rejected. They should be carefully dried in the shade. The odor is pleasant, rather aromatic, but diminishes in drying. The taste is bitter and persistent. Horehound at present brings about 1/2 to 2 cents a pound. It is well known as a domestic remedy for colds and is also used in dyspepsia and for expelling worms.

CATNIP

Nepeta cataria L.

Other common names: Cataria, catmint, catwort, catrup, field mint.

Habitat and range: Catnip, a common weed naturalized from Europe, occurs in rather dry soil in waste places and cultivated land from Canada to Minnesota and south to Virginia and Arkansas.

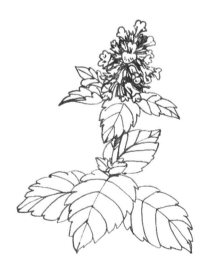

Fig. 16: Catnip

Description: The fine white hairs on the stems of this plant give it a somewhat whitish appearance. Catnip reaches about 2 to 3 feet in height, with erect, square, and branched stems. It is a perennial belonging to the mint family (Menthaceae). The opposite leaves are heart shaped or oblong, with a pointed apex, the upper surface green, the lower grayish green with fine white hairs, the margins finely scalloped and 1 to 21/2 inches in length. About June to September the many-flowered, rather thick spikes are produced at the ends of the stem and branches. The whitish flowers, dotted with purple, are two lipped, the upper lip notched or two cleft, the lower one with three lobes, the middle lobe broadest and sometimes two cleft. (Fig. 16).

Collection, prices, and uses: The leaves and flowering tops, which have a strong odor and a bitter taste, are collected when the plant is in flower and are carefully dried. The coarser stems and branches should be rejected. Catnip was official in the United States Pharmacopoeia from 1840 to 1880. The price ranges from 3 to 5 cents a pound. Catnip is used as a mild stimulant and tonic and as an emmenagogue. It also has a quieting effect on the nervous system.

MOTHERWORT

Leonurus cardiaca L.

Synonym: Cardiaca vulgaris Moench.

Other common names: Throwwort, cowthwort, lion's-tail, lion's-ear.

Habitat and range: Motherwort, naturalized from Europe and a native also of Asia, is found about dwellings and in waste places, its range in this country extending from Nova Scotia to

North Carolina, Minnesota, and Nebraska.

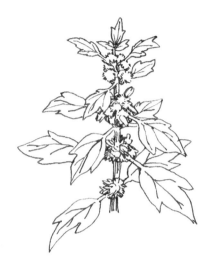

Fig. 17: Motherwort

Description: The rather stout, erect, 4-angled stem of this perennial herb attains a height of from 2 to 5 feet, is sparingly hairy, and has upright branches. The rough, dark-green leaves are borne on long stems, the lower ones rounded, about 2 to 4 inches wide and three to five lobed, the lobes pointed, toothed, or variously cut, the upper narrower ones three cleft with lance-shaped lobes. Motherwort flowers in summer, the pale-purple or pinkish lip-shaped blossoms produced in the axils of the leaves being arranged in dense circles around the stem; the upper lip is densely covered with white, woolly hairs on the outside and the lower lip is three lobed and mottled. (Fig. 17.) Motherwort belongs to the mint family (Menthaceae).

Collection, prices, and uses: The leaves and flowering tops are collected during the flowering season. They have an aromatic odor and a very bitter taste. At present they bring about 3 to 5 cents a pound. Motherwort has stimulant, slightly tonic properties and is used also to promote perspiration.

PENNYROYAL

Hedeoma. pulegioides (L.) Pers

Pharmacopoeial name: Hedeoma.

Other common names: American pennyroyal, mock pennyroyal, squaw mint, tick-weed, stinking balm, mosquito plant.

Habitat and range: Pennyroyal is found in dry soil from Nova Scotia and Quebec to Dakota and southward.

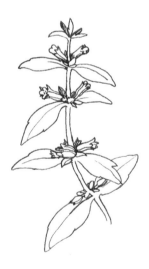

Fig. 18: Pennyroyal

Description: This very strongly aromatic annual of the mint family (Menthaceae) is of rather insignificant appearance, being a low-growing plant, about 6 inches to a foot or so in height, with a slender, erect, much-branched and somewhat hairy stem. The opposite leaves are small, scarcely exceeding three-fourths of an inch in length and becoming smaller toward the top of the plant. They are borne on short stems and are oblong ovate in shape, thin, blunt at the apex, narrowed at the base, and with margins sparingly toothed. The branchlets are four angled and somewhat hairy, and the loose flower clusters, appearing from July to September in the axils of the leaves, consist of a few pale-bluish flowers with 2-lipped corolla, the erect upper one entire or slightly notched or two lobed, while the lower spreading lip is three cleft. (Fig. 18.)

Collection, prices, and uses: The leaves and flowering tops are official in the United States Pharmacopoeia, as is also the oil of pennyroyal distilled from them. They should be collected while in flower.

The price paid to collectors ranges from about 11/4 to 21/2 cents a pound. Pennyroyal has a strong mint-like odor and pungent taste and is used as an aromatic stimulant, carminative, and emmenagogue. The odor is very repulsive to insects, and pennyroyal is therefore much used for keeping away mosquitoes and other troublesome insects.

BUGLEWEED

Lycopus virginicus L.

Other common names: Buglewort, sweet bugleweed, American water horehound, carpenter's herb, green archangel, gypsyweed, Paul's betony, wood betony, wolf foot, purple archangel, water bugle, gypsywort, gypsy herb, Virginia horehound.

Habitat and range: Bugleweed is a native herb

frequenting wet, shady places from Canada to Florida, Missouri, and Nebraska.

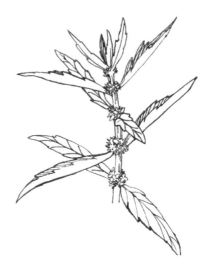

Fig. 19: Bugleweed

Description: This perennial herb of the mint family (Menthacese) has long, threadlike runners and a bluntly 4-angled, smooth, slender, erect or ascending stem from 6 inches to 2 feet in height. The leaves are dark green or of a purplish tinge, about 2 inches in length, long pointed at the apex and narrowed toward the base, the upper portion of the margin being toothed. The small, tubular, bell-shaped, 4-lobed flowers are purplish and are produced from about. July to September They are borne in dense clusters in the axils of the leaves and are followed by 3-sided nutlets. (Fig. 19.)

Collection, prices, and uses: The entire herb, which was official from 1830 to 1880, should be gathered during the flowering period. It brings about 3 to 4 cents a pound. The plant has a rather pleasant, mint-like odor, but the taste is bitter and disagreeable. It has sedative, tonic, and astringent properties.

PEPPERMINT

Mentha piperita L.

Pharmacopoeial name: Mentha piperita.

Other common names: American mint, brandy mint, lamb mint, lammint, State mint (in New York).

Habitat and range: Peppermint is naturalized from Europe and is found in damp places from Nova Scotia to Minnesota and south to Florida and Tennessee. It is largely cultivated, principally in Michigan and New York, where the distillation of the plants for the oil is carried on commercially on a very extensive scale, and also in parts of Indiana, Iowa, and Wisconsin.

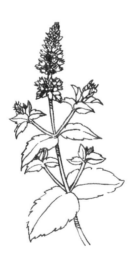

Fig. 20: Peppermint

Description: Pepper-mint propagates by means of its

long, running roots, from which are produced smooth, square stems, from 1 to 3 feet in height, erect and branching. The dark-green leaves arc borne on stalks and are lance shaped, 1 to 2 inches in length and about half as wide, pointed at the apex and rounded or narrowed at the base, with margins sharply toothed; they are smooth on both sides, or sometimes the veins on the lower surface are hairy. This aromatic perennial of the mint family (Menthaceae) is in flower from July to September, the small purplish blossoms having a tubular, 5-toothed calyx and a 4-lobed corolla. They are placed in circles around the stem, forming thick, blunt, terminal spikes. (Fig. 20.)

Collection, prices, and uses: The dried leaves and flowering tops are the parts directed to be used by the United States Pharmacopoeia. These must be collected as soon as the flowers begin to open and should be carefully dried in the shade. Dried peppermint leaves and tops bring about 31/2 to 41/2 cents a pound. The pungent odor of peppermint is familiar, as is likewise the agreeable taste, burning at first and followed by a feeling of coolness in the mouth. It is a well-known remedy for stomach and intestinal troubles. The oil, which is obtained by distillation with water from the fresh or partially dried leaves and flowering tops, is also official in the United States Pharmacopoeia. While a less acreage was devoted to peppermint during 1910, conditions were favorable to its growth, and the crop is estimated to have amounted to about 200,000 pounds. The wholesale quotations for peppermint oil in the spring of 1911 ranged from $2.85 to $2.95 a pound.

SPEARMINT

Mentha spicata L.

Pharmacopoeial name: Menthas viridis.

Synonym: Mentha viridis L.

Other common names: Mint, brown mint, garden mint, lamb mint, mackerel mint, Our Lady's mint, sage of Bethlehem.

Habitat and range: Like peppermint, the spearmint has also been naturalized from Europe and may be found in moist fields and waste places from Nova Scotia to Utah and south to Florida. It is also cultivated to some extent for the distillation of the oil and is a familiar plant in gardens for domestic use.

Description: Spearmint very much resembles peppermint. It does not grow perhaps quite so tall, the lance-shaped leaves are generally stemless or at least with very short stems, and the flowering spikes are narrow and pointed instead of thick and blunt. (Fig. 21.) The flowering period is the same as for peppermint- from July to September.

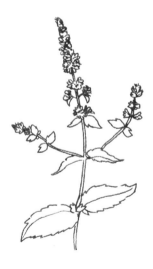

Fig. 21: Spearmint

Collection, prices, and uses: The dried leaves and flowering tops are official in the United States Pharmacopoeia and should be collected before the flowers are fully developed.

The price at present is about 3 1/2 cents a pound. Spearmint is used for similar purposes as peppermint, although its action is milder. The odor and taste closely resemble those of peppermint, but a difference may be detected, the flavor of spearmint being by some regarded as more agreeable. Oil of spearmint is also official in the United States Pharmacopoeia. It is obtained from the fresh or partially dried leaves and flowering tops.

JIMSON WEED

Datura stramonium L.

Pharmacopoeial name: Stramonium.

Other common names: Jamestown weed (from which the name "jimson weed" is derived), Jamestown lily, thorn apple, devil's apple, mad-apple, apple of Peru, stinkweed, stinkwort, devil's-trumpet, fireweed, dewtry.

Habitat and range: This is a very common weed in fields and waste places almost everywhere in the United States except in the North and West. It is widely scattered in nearly all warm countries.

Description: Jimson weed is an ill-scented, poisonous annual belonging to the nightshade family (Solanaceae). Its stout, yellowish-green stems are about 2 to 5 feet high, much forked, and leafy with large, thin, wavy-toothed leaves. The leaves are from 3 to 8 inches long, thin, smooth, pointed at the top and usually narrowed at the base, somewhat lobed or irregularly toothed and waved, veiny, the upper surface dark green, while the lower surface is a lighter green. The flowers are large (about 3 inches in length), white, funnel shaped, rather showy, and with a pronounced odor. Jimson weed is in flower from about May to September, and the seed pods which follow are dry, oval, prickly capsules, about as large as a horse-chestnut, which upon ripening burst open into four valves containing numerous black, wrinkled, kidney-shaped seeds, which are poisonous. (Fig. 22.)

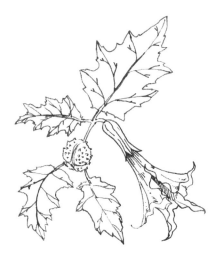

Fig. 22 Jimson Weed

Collection, prices, and uses: The leaves of the jimson weed, yielding, when assayed by the United States Pharmacopoeia process, not less than 0.35 per cent of its alkaloids, are official under the name "Stramonium." They are collected at the time jimson weed is in flower, the entire plant being cut or pulled up and the leaves stripped and carefully dried in the shade. They have an unpleasant, narcotic odor and a bitter, nauseous taste. Drying diminishes the disagreeable odor. The collector may receive from 2 to 5 cents a pound for the leaves. The leaves, which are poisonous, cause dilation of the pupil of the eye and also have narcotic, antispasmodic, anodyne, and diuretic properties. In asthma they are frequently employed in the form of cigarettes, which are smoked, or the fumes are inhaled. The seeds are also used in medicine.

BALMONY

Chelone glabra L.

Other common names: Turtlehead, turtle bloom, fishmouth, codhead, salt-rheum weed, snake-head, bitter herb, shell flower.

Habitat and range: This native perennial grows in swamps and along streams from Newfoundland to Manitoba and south to Florida and Kansas.

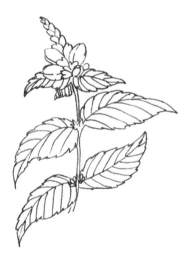

Fig. 23: Balmony

Description: Balmony is a slender, erect herb, with a 4-angled stem 1 to 3 feet in height, occasionally branched. The short-stemmed leaves, which are from 3 to 6 inches in length, are narrowly lance shaped to broadly lance shaped, the lower ones sometimes broadly oval, narrowing toward the base and with margins furnished with sharp, close-lying teeth. In late summer or early fall the showy clusters of whitish or pinkish flowers are produced. Each flower is about an inch in length, with a tubular, inflated corolla, with the mouth slightly open and resembling the head of a turtle or snake; its broad arched upper lip is keeled in the center and notched at the apex, while the lower lip is three lobed, the smallest lobe in the center, and the throat bearded with woolly hairs. (Fig. 23.) The seed capsule is oval, about half an inch in length, and contains numerous small seeds.

Collection, prices, and uses: The herb (especially the leaves), which brings from 3 to 4 cents a pound, should be collected during the flowering period. Balmony has a very bitter taste, but no odor, and is used as a tonic, for its cathartic properties, and for expelling worms.

COMMON SPEEDWELL

Veronica officinalis L.

Other common names: Paul's betony, ground-hele, fluellin, upland speedwell.

Habitat and range: This little herb frequents dry fields and woods from Nova Scotia to Michigan and south to North Carolina and Tennessee. It also occurs in Europe and Asia.

Description: The common speedwell creeps over the ground by means of rather woody stems rooting at the joints and sends up branches from 3 to 10 inches in height. It is hairy all over. The leaves are opposite to each other on the stem, on short stalks, grayish green and soft hairy, oblong or oval in shape, and about one-half to an inch in length; they are blunt at the apex, with margins saw toothed and narrowing into the stalks. From about May to July the elongated, narrow, spike-like flower clusters are produced from the leaf axils, crowded with small, pale-blue flowers. (Fig-24.) The capsule is obovate, triangular, and compressed, and contains numerous flat seeds. The speedwell is a perennial belonging to the figwort family (Scrophulariaceae).

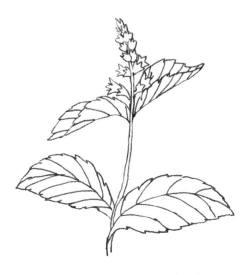

Fig. 24: Common Speedwell

Collection, prices, and uses: The leaves and flowering tops, which bring about 3 to 5 cents a pound, should be collected about May or June. When fresh they have a faint, agreeable odor, which is lacking when dry. The taste is bitter and aromatic and somewhat astringent. Speedwell has been used for asthmatic troubles and coughs and also for its alterative, tonic, and diuretic properties.

FOXGLOVE

Digitalis purpurea L.

Pharmacopoeial name: Digitalis.

Other common names: Purple foxglove, thimbles, fairy cap, fairy thimbles, fairy fingers, fairy bells, dog's-finger, finger flower, lady's-glove, lady's finger, lady's-thimble, popdock, flap dock, flop dock, lion's-mouth, rabbit's-flower, cottagers, throatwort, Scotch mercury.

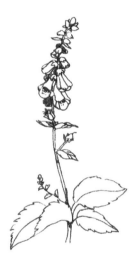

Fig. 25: Foxglove

Habitat and range: Originally introduced into this country from Europe as an ornamental garden plant, foxglove may now be found wild in a few localities in parts of Oregon, Washington, and West Virginia, having escaped from cultivation and assumed the character of a weed. It occurs along roads and fence rows, in small cleared places, and on the borders of timber land.

Description: Foxglove, a biennial or perennial belonging to the figwort family (Scrophulariaceae), during the first year of its growth produces only a dense rosette of leaves, but in the second season the downy and leafy flowering stalk, reaching a height of 3 to 4 feet, appears. The basal leaves are rather large, with long stalks, while the upper ones gradually become smaller and are borne on shorter leafstalks. The ovate or oval leaves, 4 to 12 inches long and about half as wide, the upper surface of which is dull green and wrinkled, are narrowed at the base into long winged stalks; the lower surface of the leaves shows a thick network of prominent veins and is grayish, with soft, short hairs. The apex is blunt or pointed and the margins are round toothed. When foxglove is in flower, about June, it is a most handsome plant, the long terminal clusters (about 14 inches in length) of numerous tubular, bell-shaped flowers making a very showy appearance. The individual flowers are about 2 inches long and vary in color from whitish through lavender and purple; the inside of the lower lobe is white, with crimson spots and furnished with long, soft, white hairs. (Fig. 25.) The capsule is ovoid, two celled, and many seeded.

Collection, prices, and uses: The leaves, which are official in the United States Pharmacopoeia, are collected from plants of the second year's growth just about the time that they are coming into flower. They should be very carefully dried in the shade soon after collection and as rapidly as possible, preserving them in dark, airtight receptacles. The leaves soon lose their medicinal properties if not properly dried or if exposed to light and moisture. Foxglove brings about 6 to 8 cents a pound. At present most of the foxglove or digitalis used comes to this country from Europe, where the plant grows wild and is also cultivated.

Foxglove has a faint, rather peculiar odor and a very bitter, nauseous taste. Preparations made from it are of great value in affections of the heart, but they are poisonous and should be used only on the advice of a physician.

SQUAW VINE

Mitchella repens L.

Other common names: Checkerberry, partridgeberry, deerberry, hive vine, squaw-berry, twinberry, chickenberry, cowberry, boxberry, foxberry, partridge vine, winter clover, wild running box, oneberry, pigeonberry, snakeberry, two-eyed berry, squaw-plum.

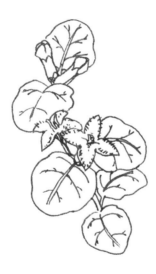

Fig. 26: Squaw Vine

Habitat and range: The squaw vine is common in woods from Nova Scotia to Minnesota and south to Florida and Arkansas, where it is generally found creeping about the bases of trees.

Description: This slender, creeping or trailing evergreen herb, a member of the madder family (Rubiaceae), has stems 6 to 12 inches long, rooting at the joints, and roundish-oval, rather

49

thick, shining, dark green opposite leaves about half an inch in length, which are blunt at the apex and rounded or somewhat heart shaped at the base, with margins entire. Sometimes the leaves show whitish veins. The plant flowers from about April to June, producing fragrant whitish, sometimes pale-purplish, funnel-shaped and 4-lobed flowers, two borne together on a stalk and having the ovaries (seed-bearing portion) united, resulting in a double, berry like fruit. These fruits are red and contain eight small, bony nutlets. (Fig. 26.) They remain on the vine through the winter and are edible, though practically tasteless.

Collection, prices, and uses: The leaves and stems (herb) are collected at almost any time of the year and range in price from about 3 1/2 to 4 cents a pound. The leaves have no odor and are somewhat astringent and bitter. Squaw vine has tonic, astringent, and diuretic properties.

LOBELIA

Lobelia inflata L.

Pharmacopoeial name: Lobelia.

Other common names: Indian tobacco, wild tobacco, asthma weed, gagroot, vomit-wort, puke weed, emetic herb, bladder pod, low belia, eyebright.

Habitat and range: Lobelia may be found in sunny situations in open woodlands, old fields and pastures, and along roadsides nearly everywhere in the United States, but especially east of the Mississippi River.

Description: This poisonous plant, an annual belonging to the bellflower family (Campanulaceae), contains an acrid, milky juice. Its simple stem has but few short branches and is smooth above, while the lower part is rough hairy. The leaves are placed alternately along the stem, those on the upper portion small and stemless and the lower leaves larger and borne on stalks. They are pale green and thin in texture, from 1 to about 2 inches in length, oblong or oval, blunt at the apex, the margins irregularly saw toothed, and both upper and lower surfaces furnished with short hairs. Lobelia may be found in flower from summer until frost, but its pale-blue flowers, while very numerous, are very small and inconspicuous. They are borne on very short stems in the axils of the upper leaves. The lower lip of each flower has three lobes and the upper one two segments, from the center of which the tube is cleft to the base. The inflated capsules are nearly round, marked with parallel grooves, and contain very numerous extremely minute dark-brown seeds. (Fig. 27.)

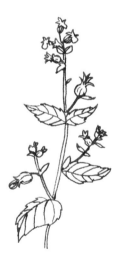

Fig. 27: Lobelia

Collection, prices, and uses: The Pharmacopoeia directs that the leaves and tops be collected after some of the capsules have become inflated. Not too much of the stemmy portion should be included. The leaves and tops should be dried in the shade and when dry kept in covered receptacles. The price paid for the dried leaves and tops is about 3 cents a pound. Lobelia has expectorant properties, acts upon the nervous system and bowels, causes vomiting, and is poisonous. The seed of lobelia is also employed in medicine.

BONESET

Eupatorium perfoliatum L.

Pharmacopoeial name: Eupatorium.

Synonym: Eupatorium connatum Michx.

Other common names: Thoroughwort, thorough-stem, thorough-wax, wood boneset, teasel, agueweed, feverwort, sweating plant, crosswort, vegetable antimony, Indian sage, wild sage, tearal, wild Isaac.

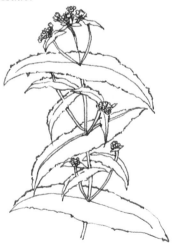

Fig. 28: Boneset

AMERICAN MEDICINAL LEAVES AND HERBS

Habitat and range: Boneset is a common weed in low, wet ground, along streams, and on the edges of swamps and in thickets from Canada to Florida and west to Texas and Nebraska.

Description: This plant is easily recognized by the peculiar arrangement of the leaves, which are opposite to each other, but joined together at the base, which makes it appear as though they were one, with the stem passing through the center. It is a perennial plant belonging to the aster family (Asteraceae), and is erect, growing rather tall, from 1 to 5 feet in height. The stout stems are rough hairy,and the leaves,united at the base, are rough, very prominently veined, wrinkled, dark green above, lighter green and downy beneath, lance shaped, tapering to a point, and with bluntly toothed margins. The crowded, flat-topped clusters of flowers are produced from about July to September and consist of numerous white tubular flowers united in dense heads. (Fig. 28.)

Collection, prices, and uses: The leaves and flowering tops, official in the United States Pharmacopoeia, are collected when the plants are in flower, stripped from the stalk, and carefully dried. They lose considerable of their weight in drying. The price per pound for boneset is about 2 cents. Boneset leaves and tops have a bitter, astringent taste and a slightly aromatic odor. They form an old and popular remedy in the treatment of fever and ague, as implied by some of the common names given to the plant. Boneset is also employed in colds, dyspepsia, jaundice, and as a tonic. In large doses it acts as an emetic and cathartic.

GUM PLANT

(1) Grindelia robusta Nutt.; (2) Grindelia squarrosa (Pursh) Dunal.

Pharmacopoeial name: Grindelia.

Other common names: (2) Broad-leaved gum plant, scaly grindelia.

Habitat and range: The gum plant (Grindelia robusta) occurs in the States west of the Rocky Mountains, while the broad leaved gum plant (G. squarrosa) is more widely distributed, being of common occurrence on the plains and prairies from the Saskatchewan to Minnesota, south to Texas and Mexico, and westward to California.

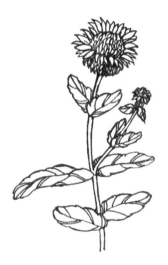

Fig. 29: Gum Plant

Description: The name "gum plant" is applied especially to Grindelia robusta on account of the fact that the entire plant is covered with a resinous substance, giving it a gummy, varnished appearance. It is an erect perennial herb belonging to the aster family (Asteraceae) and has a round smooth stem, about 11/2 feet in height. The leaves are pale green, leathery in texture and rather rigid, coated with resin and showing numerous translucent dots, and are about an inch in length. In outline they are oblong spatulate- that is, having a broad, rounded top gradually narrowing toward the base- clasping the stem and with margins somewhat saw toothed The plant branches freely near the top, each branch somewhat reddish and terminating in a large yellow flower. The yellow flowers are about three-fourths of an inch in diameter, broader than long, and are borne singly at the ends of the branches.

Immediately beneath the flower is a set of numerous, thick, overlapping scales (the involucre), the tips of which are rolled forward, the whole heavily coated with resin. The broad-leaved gum plant (Grindelia squarrosa) is very similar to G. robusta, except that it is smaller and less gummy in appearance. It is more sparingly branched near the top and the branches seem more reddish. The leaves are also clasping, but they are longer, about 2 inches in length, and broader, thinner in texture and not rigid, and more prominently toothed. The smaller flower heads are generally longer than broad and have narrower involucral scales, the recurved tips of which are longer and more slender. (Fig. 29.)

Collection, prices, and uses: The leaves and flowering tops of both species of Grindelia are official in the United States Pharmacopoeia, and should be collected about the time that the flowers have come into full bloom. The price ranges from about 5 to 10 cents a pound. While both species are official, the leaves and tops of Grindelia squarrosa, being more prevalent, are generally used. The odor of grindelia is balsamic and the taste resinous, sharply aromatic, and slightly bitter. The drug is sometimes used in asthmatic and similar affections, as a stomachic, tonic, and externally in cases of poisoning by poison ivy.

CANADA FLEABANE

Conyza canadense (L.) Britton.

Synonym: Erigeron canadensis L.

Other common names: Erigeron, horseweed, mare's-tail, Canada erigeron, butterweed, bitter-weed, cow's-tail, colt's-tail, fireweed, bloodstanch, hogweed, prideweed, scabious.

Habitat and range: Canada fleabane is common in fields and waste places and along roadsides almost throughout North America. It is also widely distributed as a weed in the Old World and in South America.

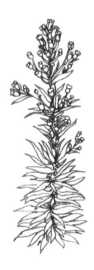

Fig. 30: Canada Fleabane

Description: The size of this weed, which is an annual, depends upon the kind of soil in which it grows, the height varying from a few inches only to sometimes 10 feet in favorable soil. The erect stem is bristly hairy or sometimes smooth, and in the larger plants usually branched near the top. The leaves are usually somewhat hairy, the lower ones 1 to 4 inches long, broader at the top and narrowing toward the base, with margins toothed, lobed, or unbroken, while those scattered along the stem are rather narrow with margins generally entire. This weed, which belongs to the aster family (Asteraceae), produces from June to November numerous heads of small, inconspicuous white flowers, followed by an abundance of seed. (Fig. 30.)

Collection, prices, and uses: The entire herb is used; it should be collected during the flowering period and carefully dried. The price paid is about 5 to 6 cents a pound. By distillation of the fresh flowering herb a volatile oil is obtained, known as oil of fleabane or oil of erigeron, which is sometimes employed in attempting to control hemorrhages and diarrheal affections. The leaves and tops were formerly official in the United States Pharmacopoeia, from 1820 to 1880, but the oil alone is now recognized as official. The herb, which has a faint agreeable odor and an astringent and bitter taste, is also used for hemorrhages from various sources and the bleeding of wounds. It is also employed in diarrhea and dropsy.

YARROW

Achillea millefolium L.

Other common names: Millefolium, milfoil, thousand-leaf, thousandleaf clover, gordolobo, green arrow, soldier's wound-wort, nosebleed, dog daisy, bloodwort, sanguinary, carpenter's grass, old-man's-pepper, cammock.

Habitat and range: Yarrow is very common along roadsides and in old fields, pastures, and meadows from the New England States to Missouri and in scattered localities in other parts of the country.

Description: This weed, a perennial of the aster family (Asteraceae), is about 10 to 20 inches in height and has many dark-green feathery leaves, narrowly oblong or lance shaped in outline and very finely divided into numerous crowded parts or segments. Some of the leaves, especially the basal ones, which are borne on stems, are as much as 10 inches in length and about half an inch or an inch in width. The leaves toward the top of the plant become smaller and stemless. From about June to September the flat-topped flowering heads are produced in abundance and consist of numerous small, white (sometimes rose-colored), densely crowded flowers. (Fig. 31.) Yarrow has a strong odor, and when it is eaten by cows the odor and bitter taste are transmitted to dairy products.

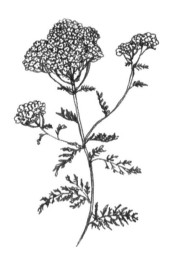

Fig. 31: Yarrow

Collection, prices, and uses: The entire plant is collected at the time that it is in flower and is carefully dried. The coarser stems are rejected. Considerable shrinkage takes place in drying, the plant losing about four-fifths of its weight. The prices paid for yarrow are from about 3 to 5 cents a pound. Yarrow was official in the United States Pharmacopoeia from 1860 to 1880. It has a strong, aromatic odor, very much like chamomile, and a sharp, bitter taste. It has been used as a stimulant tonic, for its action upon the bladder, and for checking excessive discharges.

TANSY

Tanacetum vulgare L.

Other common name: Tanacetum, bitter buttons, ginger plant, parsley fern. scented fern, English cost, hindheal.

Habitat and range: This is another garden plant introduced into this country from Europe and now escaped from cultivation, occurring as a weed along waysides and fences from New England to Minnesota and southward to North Carolina and Missouri.

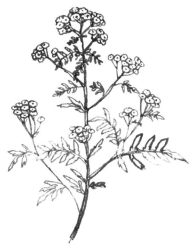

Fig. 32: Tansy

Description: Tansy is strong-scented perennial herb with finely divided, fern-like leaves and yellow button-like flowers, and belongs to the aster family (Asteraceae). It has a stout, somewhat reddish, erect stem, usually smooth, 11/2 to 3 feet high, and branching near the top. The entire leaf is about 6 inches long, its general outline oval, but it is divided nearly to the midrib into about seven pairs of segments, or lobes, which like the terminal one are again divided for about two thirds of the distance to the midvein into smaller lobes having saw-toothed margins, giving to the leaf a somewhat feathery or fern-like appearance. The yellow flowers, borne in terminal clusters, are roundish and flat topped, surrounded by a set of dry, overlapping scales (the involucre). (Fig. 32.) Tansy is in flower from about July to September.

Collection, prices, and uses: The leaves and flowering tops of tansy are collected at the time of flowering and are carefully dried. They lose about four-fifths of their weight in drying. Their price ranges from about 3 to 5 cents a pound. Tansy has a strong, aromatic odor and a bitter taste. It is poisonous and has been known to produce fatal results. It has stimulant, tonic, and emmenagogue properties and is also used as a remedy against worms.

WORMWOOD

Artemisia absinthium L.

Synonym: Artemisia vulgaris Lam.

Other common names: Absinthium, absinth, madderwort, mingwort, old-woman, warmot, mugwort.

Habitat and range: Wormwood, naturalized from Europe and mostly escaped from gardens in this country, is found in waste places and along roadsides from Newfoundland to New York and westward. It is occasionally cultivated.

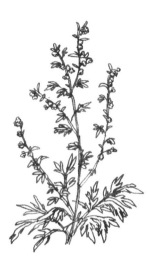

Fig. 33: Wormwood

Description: This shrubby, aromatic, much-branched perennial of the aster family (Asteraceae) is from 2 to 4 feet in height, hoary, the young shoots silvery white with fine silky hairs. The grayish-green leaves are from 2 to 5 inches long, the lower long-stalked ones two to three times divided into leaflets with lance-shaped lobes, the upper leaves gradually becoming more simple and stemless and borne on short stems and the uppermost linear with unbroken margins. The flower clusters, appearing from July to October, consist of numerous small, insignificant, drooping, flat-globular, yellow heads. (Fig.33.)

Collection, prices, and uses: When the plant is in flower the leaves and flowering tops are collected. These were official in the United States Pharmacopoeia for 1890. The price paid for wormwood is about 4 cents a pound. Wormwood has an aromatic odor and an exceedingly bitter taste, and is used as a tonic, stomachic, stimulant, against fevers, and for expelling worms. An oil is obtained from wormwood by distillation which is the main ingredient in the dangerous liqueur known as absinth, long a popular drink in France, in which country, however, the use of the oil is now prohibited except by pharmacists in making up prescriptions.

COLTSFOOT

Tussilago farfara L.

Other common names: Coughwort, assfoot, horsefoot, foalfoot, bull'sfoot, horsehoof, colt-herb, clayweed, cleats, dovedock, dummyweed, ginger, gingerroot, hoofs, sowfoot, British tobacco, gowan.

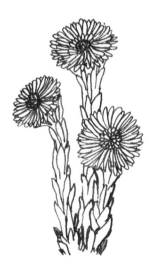

Fig. 34: Coltsfoot

Habitat and range: Coltsfoot has been naturalized in this country from Europe, and is found along brooks and in wet places and moist clayey soil along roadsides from Nova Scotia and New Brunswick to Massachusetts, New York, and Minnesota.

Description: In spring the white-woolly, scaly flowering stalks with their yellow blossoms are the first to appear, the leaves not being produced until the seed has formed or at least toward the latter part of the flowering stage. The flowering stalks are several, arising from the root, and are from 3 to 18 inches in height, each one bearing at the top a single, large yellow head, reminding one of a dandelion, having in the center what are called disk flowers, which are tubular, and surrounded by what are known as ray flowers, which are strap shaped. When the seed is ripe the head looks somewhat like a dandelion "blow." The flowering heads are erect, after flowering nodding, and again erect in fruit. The bright-yellow flowers only open in sunshiny weather. They have a honeylike odor.

The leaves, as already stated, appear when the flowers are almost through blossoming, or even afterwards. They are large, 3 to 7 inches wide, almost round or heart shaped in outline, or, according to some of the names applied to it, shaped like a horse's hoof; the margins are slightly lobed and sharply toothed. The upper surface is smooth and green, while the lower is white with densely matted woolly hairs. All the leaves arise from the root and are borne on long, erect stalks. (Fig. 34.)

Collection, prices, and uses: All parts of coltsfoot are active, but the leaves are mostly employed; they should be collected in June or July, or about the time when they are nearly full size. When dry, they break very readily. Collectors are paid about 31/2 cents a pound. Coltsfoot leaves form a popular remedy in coughs and other affections of the chest and throat, having a soothing effect on irritated mucous membranes. The flowers are also used; likewise the root.

FIREWEED

Erechthites hieracifolia (L.) Raf.

Synonym: Senecio hieracifolius L.

Another common name: Pilewort.

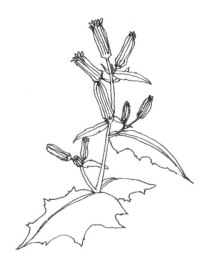

Fig. 35: Fireweed

Habitat and range: Fireweed is found in woods, fields, and waste places from Canada to Florida, Louisiana, and Nebraska, springing up in especial abundance where land has been burned over, whence the name "fire-weed."

Description: This weed is a native of this country and is an ill-smelling annual belonging to the aster family (Asteraceae). The stem is from 1 to 8 feet in height, grooved, branched, and juicy. The light green leaves are rather large, from 2 to 8 inches long, thin in texture, lance shaped or oval lance shaped, the margins toothed or sometimes deeply cut. The upper ones usually have a clasping base or are at least stemless, while the margins of those lower down narrow into the stems.

Fireweed is in flower from about July to September, the flat-topped clusters of greenish-white or whitish heads being produced from the ends of the stem and branches. The green outer covering of each flower head is cylindrical, with the base considerably swollen. (Fig. 35.) The seed is furnished with numerous soft white bristles.

Collection, prices, and uses: The entire plant is used and is gathered in summer. The leaves turn black in drying. The price paid to collectors ranges from about 2 to 3 cents a pound. An oil is obtained by distillation from the fresh plant. Fireweed has a disagreeable taste and odor. It has astringent, tonic, and alterative properties.

BLESSED THISTLE

Cnicus benedictus L.

Synonyms: Centaurea benedicta L.; Carduus benedictus Cam.; Carbenia benedicta Adans.

Other common names: Holy thistle, St. Benedict's thistle, Our Lady's thistle, bitter thistle, spotted thistle, cursed thistle, blessed cardus, spotted cardus.

Habitat and range: The blessed thistle is a weed which has been introduced into this country from southern Europe and is found in waste places and stony, uncultivated localities from Nova Scotia to Maryland and the Southern States; also on the Pacific coast. It is cultivated in many parts of Europe.

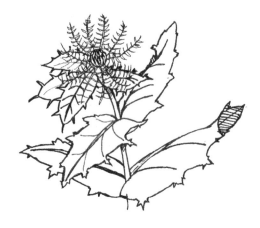

Fig. 36: Blessed Thistle

Description: In height this annual plant of the aster family (Asteraceae) scarcely exceeds 2 feet, with coarse erect stems, branched and rather woolly. The leaves are large, 3 to 6 inches long or more, oblong lance shaped, thin, more or less hairy, with margins wavy lobed and spiny. The lower leaves and those at the bottom are narrowed toward the base into winged stems, while those near the top are stemless and clasping.

The yellow flower heads, which appear from about May to August, are situated at the ends of the branches, almost hidden by the upper leaves, and are about an inch and a half in length. Immediately surrounding the yellow flower heads are scales of a leathery texture, tipped with- long, hard, branching, yellowish-red spines. (Fig. 36.)

Collection, prices, and uses: The leafy flowering tops and the other leaves are gathered preferably just before or during the blossoming period and then are thoroughly and quickly dried. In the fresh state the leaves and tops have a rather disagreeable odor, which they lose on drying. They are bright green when fresh and grayish green and woolly when dry. Collectors receive about 6 to 8 cents a pound. The taste of the blessed thistle is very bitter and salty and somewhat acrid. It, is used principally as a bitter tonic.

THE END

Made in the USA
Monee, IL
13 May 2023